GABOR PALOS

SIMPLIFIED BALBOA FOR MEN

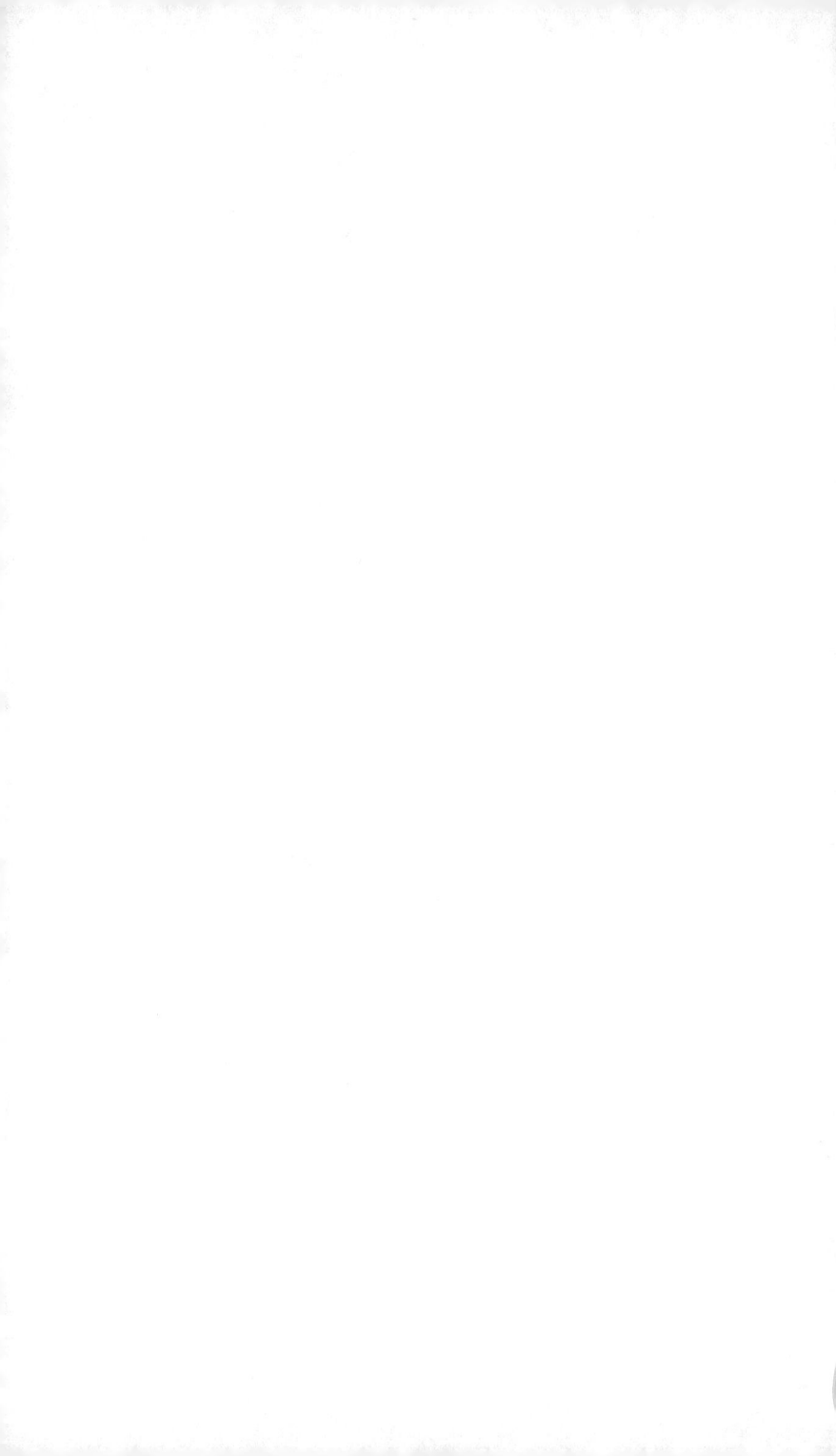

Gabor Palos

Simplified Balboa
for Men

GABOR PALOS

SIMPLIFIED BALBOA FOR MEN

First Edition 2024

ISBN 978-1-7770046-3-7

Table of Contents

Introduction

This book is a guide for those wanting to learn the leader's part of the fast and smooth swing dance called Balboa.

It is intended to put the reader on the dance floor as soon as possible, therefore it will focus on basic background information and the most important steps of the dance.

While Lindy Hop is the most popular swing dance which is best danced to medium tempo music, Balboa is a most excellent dance for fast swing music. Lindy Hop and Balboa pair very well and, together, cover a wide range of tempos.

For such a beautiful and practical dance, not much has been written about Balboa. The aim of this book is to fill this gap and to be simple and practical.

Enjoy learning and dancing the Balboa!

May 2024

About Balboa

The swing dance called Balboa originated in Southern California in the 1930s and is said to be named after the Balboa Pavilion in Newport Beach.

The pavilion was built on a seaside pier as a boat house on the Balboa Peninsula in the early 20th century. During the 1930s it served as a dance hall and featured famous jazz big bands and hosted large swing dance parties. This is when the dance Balboa was born.

After World War II, the Balboa Pavilion served various other purposes and it still stands as a historic landmark.

The new dance was very popular in the 1930s and 40s on the West Coast and even produced a few outstanding professional dancers. It was featured in a short clip in the 1938 Hollywood movie "Start Cheering". Another contemporary video recording of swing dancing, including some Balboa steps, was filmed on Venice Beach, California around the same time.

Following World War II, the popularity of social dancing gradually declined and Balboa faded into obscurity until it was re-discovered in the 1980s.

Today Balboa enjoys a renewed interest all over the world and group classes teaching Balboa are relatively easy to find.

<u>Styles of Balboa</u>

Balboa is a spot dance, which means that it is danced in one spot, and a swing dance, which means that it was meant to be danced to

3

swing music. Swing was the most popular type of jazz music in the 1930s and 40s, played by large bands in the United States.

You can find more about swing music and swing dancing in my book "Simplified Lindy Hop for Men" which also includes Lindy Hop steps and figures, Lindy Charleston steps, break or jazz steps and footwork variations, dancing to fast and slow music and tips on learning, practicing and social dancing.

We can loosely differentiate two main styles of Balboa: Pure Balboa ("Pure Bal") and Balboa Swing ("Bal Swing").

Pure Bal is also referred to as "Balboa Shuffle". It is the original version of the two styles, developed before Lindy Hop reached the West Coast. Pure Bal is danced almost exclusively in closed position, chest-to-chest in a close embrace, with most of the action taking place below the waist using elaborate footwork with small steps on a small area of the dance floor.

This character of the dance was largely the result of ballroom regulations at the time when internal migration to California led to overcrowded dance halls. Management of the Balboa Pavilion and the nearby Rendezvous Ballroom attempted to accommodate the crowds by introducing rules that included no breaking away from your partner, no wide body movements and no travelling on the dance floor. And so the popular dances of the day, One Step, Charleston and Foxtrot became stationary shuffling and morphed into what has become known as Balboa.

As Lindy Hop started to influence dancers on the West Coast, they responded by adding new elements to Balboa, incorporating steps in a more open dance position which makes various underarm turns and other fancy figures possible. Pure Bal was freed from some of its constraints and "Bal Swing" was born.

It is the Bal Swing version of Balboa that is generally taught in group classes today.

Other swing dances

The closest "living relatives" of Balboa are other swing dances like the Lindy Hop, East Coast Swing, Jitterbug, Jive, Charleston and Breakaway, the St. Louis Shag, the Collegiate Shag and Slow Balboa.

Lindy Hop is by far the most popular and most versatile swing dance that is danced socially. East Coast Swing and Jive are simplified and standardised "6-count" Ballroom versions of the Lindy Hop and as such are popular with Ballroom dancers.

Although "West Coast Swing" has "swing" in its name, it is not generally danced to swing music.

Slow Balboa is a dance that originated around the same time and at the same place as Balboa did. Slow Balboa is not exactly a slower version of Balboa (as the name would suggest) but it is closely related to it.

In contrast to most other swing dances that are generally danced to faster music, Slow Balboa is danced to slow swing music and is probably the best swing dance to reach for when the music gets too slow even for Lindy Hop. Slow Balboa is explained in more detail in my book "Simplified Slow Dancing for Men".

A fast and practical dance

Balboa is a fast, yet elegant, restrained and economical dance. It is very well suited to swing music that has a tempo in the 180-220 beats per minute (or BPM) range. This is the same tempo range as for Classic Charleston and Breakaway, so these dances are interchangeable.

Balboa is fast but it is manageable and it does not need to be exhausting because movements are relatively small and restrained. It is therefore the perfect swing dance to choose when the music gets fast.

Another feature of Balboa which makes it so well suited to fast music is that it does not have "triple-steps" like Lindy Hop does. Balboa is danced in small single steps so that it does not become frenetic as Lindy Hop can become when the music gets fast. To the onlooker, Balboa may at times look like shuffling in one place.

If one would want to describe the character of Balboa in one word, that word would be "smooth". Balboa is about smooth. "Elegant" and "sophisticated" also come to mind.

Balboa figures

It is important to remember that Balboa is a living "street dance" with no standard steps or rules and no official body or society to decide in such matters. Nothing that you will read, see or hear about the dance is cast in stone, and there is no "correct way" to dance the Balboa.

Balboa was born on the dance floor, and the figures commonly danced today are those that were handed down by a few old timers in the 1980s and 90s, each of whom remembered things from the 1930s somewhat differently, and what they did remember they did not always remember it clearly.

The original contemporary video footage of Balboa is about 25 seconds long and contain only two identifiable figures.

All this means that it doesn't pay to be too "dogmatic" about Balboa. There may have been many figures and ways of dancing the Balboa we will never know of, and new figures will certainly be invented by young dancers in the future.

The Balboa shuffle

The steps one takes in Balboa are not so much lifting the foot from the floor and putting it down.

In Balboa, keep your feet always close to the ground and slide your feet rather than stepping. The dance can also be described as "shuffling" or pushing into the ground. Hence the nickname of the dance: "Balboa Shuffle".

Basic rhythm and footwork

Compared to Lindy Hop's somewhat confusing 6- and 8-count figures, all figures in Balboa are thankfully 8-count, which means that they cover 8 beats of music, although double turns and "repetitive" type of figures may cover any (even) number of beats.

As with most swing dances, the leader starts on left foot and the follower on right foot.

The basic rhythm is an even "1-2-3-4-5-6-7-8", however both the "1-2-3-4" and the "5-6-7-8" include only three steps or weight changes. Therefore, you will dance every "1" on left foot and every "5" on right foot.

Dancing "up" and "down"

Each 4-beat half of an 8-count figure can be danced "up" or "down", according to the requirements of the particular figure. "Up" (or "up-hold") and "down" (or "down-hold") refer to where your foot is on the third beat:

- 1-2 and 5-6 are (almost) always two full steps or weight changes.

- 3-4 and 7-8 involve one step/weight change and one hold. The beat that does not have a step or weight change is a "hold", meaning that you hold your foot (in the air or on the ground) for one beat without switching your weight to it. Depending on which beat is the "step" and which beat is the "hold", each 4-beat half of the Balboa basic can be danced either "up" or "down" as follows:

  o The "up" version is: "Step-step-hold-step" (1-2-&-4)

  o The "down" version is: "Step-step-step-hold" (1-2-3-&)

Put it differently: the "up" version means that on beat 3 your foot is "up" in the air, and the "down" version means that on beat 3 your foot is "down" on the floor.

The "up" version is the typical Balboa footwork while the "down" version is used to facilitate certain figures.

"Up" does not mean that you should lift your foot high off the floor. Generally, Balboa is a shuffle and your foot should stay close to the floor even when it is "up".

Similarly, "hold" does not necessarily mean that the foot should be held motionless. What you do on the "hold" is a matter of style. The hold could be, among other possibilities:

- A small kick downward with the heel
- A small forward kick on 3 and a small backward kick on 7 (each pointing into the direction of the next step)
- A weightless touch-down with the ball of the foot
- A tap on the floor with the tip of the shoe next to the heel of the other shoe

- A small flick outwards with the tip of the shoe, or conversely an inward flick with the heel of the shoe

The small flick outwards with the tip of the shoe may also be added to the regular down steps as a styling element.

Learning the Balboa

For someone wanting to learn to dance the Balboa and starting it from scratch, there are several sources of information available, including group lessons, online resources, perhaps private lessons, and this book.

The benefit of reading a book like this is that the reader will have a better idea of what to expect in a group class, he will better recognize and follow what is being taught and generally have an overall prior understanding of the dance. This can be a significant boost and it could mean the difference between frustration and enjoyment, between giving up and persevering, and ultimately between learning the Balboa or not.

Group lessons are very useful for meeting and getting to know your fellow dancers, learning and practicing the basic steps, becoming part of the local dance scene, benefitting from the instructors' experience and the opportunity to dance with many followers.

Ultimately however, there is no substitute for going out, practicing and putting your skills to the test at social dances.

Reading this book, taking lessons and going out to dance should go hand-in-hand.

The steps in this book

The figures covered in this book are sufficient to provide a solid foundation. They are enough for dancing the night away with reasonable variety. If you learn to do these steps with confidence you will certainly be considered a competent dancer who knows what he is doing.

Keep in mind that the essence of swing dancing is playfulness and style. Dancing well what you know is more important than constantly learning new steps.

The entries and exits for each dance figure in this book have been chosen for illustration only. There are many other ways to enter or exit a particular figure. Finding these comes naturally after one has mastered the basics.

This book has no pictures, illustrations, or "foot charts" because they are generally tedious to make and even more difficult to follow. The goal is to provide an overview of the most important steps and describe the mechanics of each step without going into minute detail. You will no doubt also find and study these steps in group classes or in online videos.

It is important to remember that Balboa is not a standardized dance, and therefore each of these steps can go under various names and can have numerous other variations, entries and exits than those presented here.

Group classes

Group classes are very useful as entry points into the world of Balboa, and they are good for learning the basic steps and for gaining the initial experience of dancing with many followers. You should take every group class offered where you live.

Local instructors tend to be very nice people who do the teaching out of love for the dance. They are typically not professional dance instructors and do this part-time while having a day job. Their efforts should be appreciated because without them, there would be no Balboa.

At the same time, dance instruction is a difficult art and the average local Balboa teacher will typically have no training in it. The quality of instruction will vary accordingly, and group classes sometimes turn out to be less than well-structured and articulate exercises.

Teaching will generally be limited to demonstrating a figure a couple of times, then asking the class to follow, which can be difficult to do. Some aspects of a figure may be discussed, often at length, but breaking down a figure to its individual steps and leading the class through it step-by-step, which would appear to be a logical approach, seems completely and curiously absent from swing dance instruction. This means that group class students often need to be patient and do some additional research.

If you go to a group class hoping to also learn how to remember the steps shown, how to put them together in a real dance, how to start or end a dance, how to deal with mistakes and how to make your dance interesting, in most cases you might as well forget about it. Asking questions like this in class will likely draw some blank stares.

Balboa is a "street dance" without set rules, and each instructor will teach their own interpretation of it, which can be different from what other instructors teach. It is best to follow each instructor's method without questioning, and then trying them out and deciding for yourself what works best for you.

As a practical matter, beside your dance shoes, also bring a water bottle to classes, a folding fan if it is a hot day, and try to position yourself to stay away from the loudspeakers.

As useful as they are, group classes clearly have their limitations and you should not rely on them too heavily in learning to dance. Taking classes endlessly will not make one a dancer. The only place you can really learn how to dance is on the social dance floor.

Think of classes as just a bonus or an introduction, because ultimately it is up to you and no one else whether you will learn to dance or not.

Practicing

The secret to learning any dance is consistent and persistent practice. Practice comes in two forms: practicing alone or with a partner, and going to social dances as often as you can.

You absolutely should practice alone. Study a Balboa figure in detail, free up some floor space at home, and do that figure slowly, step by step, paying attention to what your feet, arms, hands, body and head are doing, and where your follower would be at any point in time.

Any dance figure is only difficult because your body is not used to that particular sequence of muscle movements. Allow your body to gradually get used to the figure. Then do it increasingly faster. Repeat it 50 and 100 times until you can do it without paying attention. Practice transitions between figures, getting into figures and exiting figures. Study and practice how to start and end a dance.

At the same time, go out and participate in social dances. The social dance floor is the best (and ultimately only) dance teacher. First practice and dance simple figures even though they may not feel too exciting, then add more figures little by little. Not going to social dances until you are sure that you have all the steps nailed down guarantees that you will never learn to dance.

Go out and practice the Balboa until it becomes second nature. You will most certainly have a lot of fun and, to be sure, you will fail a lot, too. Failure is the price of success, and trying and failing is the only way to learn, so your best option is to embrace failing as part of the process that leads to success. Don't be a perfectionist. Swallow your pride and forge ahead. There is no other way.

Swing social dance events tend to be friendly and informal affairs where most everyone is approachable and willing to dance. Having a steady dance partner has some pros and cons, and is certainly not necessary. If you do have a dance partner, then you can grow together as dancers, be familiar with each other, and therefore she will know how to follow your lead. This can be satisfying but it also means that your ability to lead others will diminish, and you will miss out on the social aspect of dancing.

Dressing to dance

When it comes to dancing, the most important piece of clothing is your shoes. Generally for dancing, comfortable, well-fitting, flexible shoes are recommended with a sole that is not sticky but not too slippery either. With Balboa however, because of the "shuffling" nature of the dance, it is okay to wear more slippery shoes.

Purpose-built dance shoes are good but often expensive and certainly not necessary. Leather soles are generally fine for dancing as long as the shoes are well broken in.

The rest of your clothing should be light and should not restrict movement. Ideal are light cotton or linen pants with a comfortable cut.

Similarly, choose shirts that are light and made of a fabric that absorbs moisture. If you dance for any length of time, you will be sweating, so choose a shirt that does not show sweat stains. Moisture absorbing polyester shirts, T-shirts or golf shirts are usually great and some are quite stylish. It is a good idea to carry a spare shirt to a dance. When you get soaked, go to the rest room and change into the spare.

Back in the day, social dancers used to dress up very nicely. These days most swing dancers dress casually when they go out to dance. This is fine, to a degree, but Balboa is an elegant, smooth dance and dressing in style will add to the fun.

Safety

Dancing is vigorous physical activity and it puts serious stress on the body. Dance at your own risk, and make sure that you are suitably fit before you start. If you have any doubts, ask your doctor for advice.

You should warm up before practice, classes or dances. Warming up is important before any physical activity and dancing is no exception.

Before attempting any step or figure, make sure that you can execute them without accidents or injuries to you, your partner or anyone else.

Shoulders and knees are particularly prone to injuries. The risk of injury to shoulder joints applies mostly to followers. If you notice that your follower is physically weak, older, or holds her arms at dangerous angles, be extra gentle with her.

Carry a water bottle and drink frequently to avoid dehydration, and stay away from the loudspeakers as the music is often unnecessarily loud.

Progress in learning

Learning to dance is a long term commitment. It is important to maintain motivation and to remember that the learning process rarely means fast or even progress, so do not get discouraged if at times you don't see any apparent improvement.

Learning often has its ups and downs and one needs to hang in there regardless. Those who do not quit and continue dancing will eventually get better and better. You need to persevere.

Having said that, sometimes it can be useful to take a temporary break from dancing, especially when focused learning and practice starts to feel like a chore. You can then return refreshed some time later with renewed energy and enthusiasm. Whatever you had already learned will have time to settle in your mind and muscles.

Posture and connection

Posture

Every style or genre of dancing has a certain basic posture that is most efficient for that particular dance, one which best accommodates and facilitates the connected movement of the dancing couple.

Balboa is an upright dance which requires both parties to stand erect, lean very slightly forward and connect at the chest or upper body.

The upright posture is maintained throughout the dance, whether in closed or open position.

Dance positions

In most dances, the two common positions of the dancers relative to each other are the open and closed position. Balboa is largely danced in closed position, with occasional separations. Pure Bal is danced in closed position exclusively.

Closed position

In closed position, the leader places his right hand on the follower's back, and takes the follower's right hand with his left hand, holding it at approximately at the level of her shoulder. The dancers are facing each other in a slightly offset position (she is somewhat to your right).

Closed dance position, in general, may or may not involve body contact. Balboa, in particular, does require body contact, the contact being chest-to-chest or belly-to-belly, the leader aiming

19

very slightly to the left, and the follower leaning and gently pressing against the right chest of the leader.

Some figures, like the Swivels, are danced in closed position but without body contact and with a small distance between the dancers to accommodate their respective movements.

For each couple, a comfortable dance position will depend on the relative body shapes and sizes and mutual comfort levels.

The frontal body-to-body connection is obviously a very intimate way of dancing. In this respect, Balboa differs from Lindy Hop which is danced mostly in open or side-by-side closed positions, and also differs from the standard or smooth ballroom dances which typically require hip-to-hip contact with the upper bodies leaning away from each other.

The posture, connection and handhold of the Balboa closed position is somewhat more similar to the close embrace of Argentine Tango.

Due to the close body connection, much of the leading is done with the upper body and not with the hands. As an exercise to get a better feel for this, put both of your hands behind your back, ask the follower to do the same, take up dance position without using hands, and try to dance a few simple Balboa figures leading with body contact only.

Open position

In open position, the dancers stand one step apart from each other and maintain only handhold or temporarily no contact at all, such as when performing a free spin. Other dance positions, such as the cuddle (or sweetheart) and the tandem position (one dancer behind the other) are not typically used in Balboa.

Handhold

In Balboa, the hand contact is almost always left-to-right (your left hand to her right hand).

In closed position, hold the follower's right hand with your left hand halfway between the two of you and at the level of her shoulder, regardless of any height difference.

Rarely, right-to-right and/or left-to-left handhold (cross-handhold or "handshake") is used, for example in the Beach Pushes or in the Texas Tommy. Also rarely, right-to-left handhold is used, for example in the Reverse Toss-Out.

Other handholds such as double handhold or double cross-hold are not typically used in Balboa.

In certain figures, the partners move away from each other creating a stretch in the handhold, or move towards each other, pressing their hands against each other creating a push or compression between the hands.

Pulsing

Swing music has a clear and characteristic rhythm, and allowing your body to "pulse" to the rhythm of the music is a characteristic feature of swing dancing.

Pulsing is moving your body down and up to the rhythm of the music. It is your inner metronome, and helps you stay in sync with the music and keep the connection between the partners.

Pulsing is done from the knee, rather than bouncing on the toes, and it is more pronounced when the music is medium tempo, such as in Lindy Hop.

Balboa is danced in an upright position, so the pulsing has to adjust to that. Since Balboa is also a fast dance, the pulsing will necessarily be quick and shallow, nevertheless it should be always present.

Basic Balboa figures

<u>The Basic Step (or Basic Box)</u>

Imagine a 1 foot by 1 foot square (or box) on the floor. This is the area in which you will be dancing the Basic Box.

Stand in the centre of the box with your weight on your right foot.

1. Step back with your left foot to the bottom left corner of the box
2. Step to the side with your right foot to the bottom right corner of the box
3. Hold your left foot
4. Step down on left foot to the centre point of the box

Now you do the mirror image in a forward direction:

5. Step forward with your right foot to the top right corner of the box
6. Step to the side with your left foot to the top left corner of the box
7. Hold your right foot
8. Step down on right foot to the centre point of the box

The 8-count sequence described above is the Basic Box danced in the more common "up" version. The "down" version would mean that you step down on 3 and 7 to the centre point of the box and keep your foot down on the following beat. Generally, however, there is no reason to use the "up" version while dancing only the Basic Box.

For variety, you can rotate gradually to the left or to the right while doing the Basic Box. If you do this, you will of course no longer step on the corners of the box.

Once you take up closed dance position with your partner and before launching into the Basic Box, it is useful to start pulsing and doing some wiggles or weight changes to the music in order to get into sync with your follower.

Balboa is a very rewarding dance because doing just this basic Balboa shuffle on a box, with gradual turns to left or right, is already fun and satisfying and can take you through a song in a pinch.

Linear Basic

This move is similar to the Basic Box but instead of dancing on a box or square, you will be dancing on a short slot moving forward and backward.

Start the Linear Basic with a "rock-step-hold-step" where you first step is back on left, forward on right, hold one beat on 3, and step forward on 4 (1-2-&-4). As an option, on the initial rock step you can lead the follower into a rock step as well (i.e. you briefly separate).

From here, you will be marching forward and backward as follows:

Forward: the next "step-step" will be two small steps forward (RF-LF), then hold on the third beat, and step back on the last beat (RF) (5-6-&-8).

Backward: the next "step-step" will be two small steps backward (LF-RF), then hold on the third beat, and step forward on the last beat (LF) (1-2-&-4).

24

Continue repeating this sequence. On 1-2, you always walk backwards and on 5-6, you always walk forward. The "hold" always starts the direction change.

The rock-step is only used to start the sequence from a standing position.

Travelling Basic

The Linear Basic can be extended either backward or forward. You simply need to skip the "hold", do not reverse direction, but rather keep marching in the same direction in closed position, in single steps. Apply the "hold" again when you want to stop and reverse direction.

In effect, the 1-2 or 5-6 ("step-step") part of the Linear Basic is extended and repeated any number of times. Between the "hold-steps" you can trot in this manner as long as you wish, either forward or backward. This can be used for variety and it is also a useful tool if you want to move to another part of the dance floor.

Walking forward (with three repeats) will be like this:
1-2-3-4-5-6-<u>5-6-5-6-5-6</u>-7-8

Walking backward (with three repeats) will be like this:
5-6-7-8-1-2-<u>1-2-1-2-1-2</u>-3-4

Lean very slightly into the direction of movement (lean forward when marching forward, lean back when marching backward).

If you do this backward, make sure no one is behind you, otherwise you may back into another couple.

Out-and-Ins

The Out-and-Ins are danced "down".

During this figure you will stop moving in sync, together in closed position, and start moving into opposite directions: away from and towards each other, mirroring each other.

Start this figure after dancing the first half of a Basic, danced "down": 1-2-down-&.

Still facing each other, you now step back on RF on 5 (instead of forward as you would normally do on 5) and she also steps back. You are now both stepping "out" or away from each other. Close your LF to RF on 6 and then step forward on 7 as she mirrors what you do. You are now both stepping "in" or coming together.

Moving "out" results in a stretch between the two of you that will bring both of you "in" again, and moving "in" results in a compression that will send both of you "out" again. Stretch-compress-stretch-compress. For this reason, the step is sometimes also referred to as Push Breaks.

Keep the back step small so that you can maintain an upright position and do not lean into each other when stepping "out".

Each Out-and-In takes 4 beats: 2 beats "out" and 2 beats "in". The footwork is "step-step-step-hold", consisting of: step back, close your other foot, step forward, hold. In 8 counts therefore there are two Out-and-Ins: on 1, you step back on left foot and on 5, you step back on right foot.

Repeat the Out-and-Ins for as long as you wish. Exit by simply easing back into the Balboa Basic, or more elegantly, turning it into a Come Around (described further below).

The Out-and-Ins are a very common, practical and often used figure that serve very well to connect other figures or used as a simple exit from many rotating figures.

Variations on the Out-and-Ins

You can add some spice to the basic Out-and-Ins and turn them into various fun figures. Here are some examples.

Rotating Out-and-Ins

Adding some circularity to an otherwise static move immediately makes it more interesting.

While doing Out-and-Ins, start gradually rotating to right. Keep turning to right over a couple of Out-and-Ins. Do your rotation mostly on the forward steps.

Now reverse the direction of the turns and rotate gradually to left over the next couple of Out-and-Ins.

Side-stepping Out-and-Ins

Instead of stepping straight-forward on 3 and 7, step as follows:
- On 3/ forward and diagonally to left on LF, and
- On 7/ forward and diagonally to right on RF

This adds a new dimension to the Out-and-Ins: the figure moves not only out and in, but also sideways left and right.

Crossovers

The "Crossovers" are a variation of the side-stepping Out-and-Ins.

Instead of stepping straight-forward on 3 and 7, step as follows:
- On 3/ forward and diagonally to right on LF, and
- On 7/ forward and diagonally to left on RF

When you step forward, turn your torso in the direction of the forward step, about 1/8 alternatingly to left and to right. She will do the same, and this will position you almost side-by-side (but facing opposite directions) on every forward step.

Similar figures are also known in other dances and may go under "Shoulder to Shoulder" or similar names.

Lazy Out-and-Ins

If you are really lazy, you can stop stepping at all. Just pulse in place and push Out (1) and pull In (3).

Scoots

"Scoots" are essentially repeated side steps into one direction, to left or to right, done in a "limping" manner.

From the Basic, step down firmly on 3, lean into it, and hold on 4. Now "Scoot" sideways to your right for 8 beats: "step-close-step-close-step-close-step-&".

Always "step" on RF, rising on the ball of your foot, then close your LF to RF, pulling it in down-flat to make the Scoots look a bit like limping. Keep your weight over your left foot throughout and lean somewhat to left (opposite the direction of the side steps).

Make the last "step" on RF (7) a strong down-step and transfer your weight to RF. Hold the next beat. For variety, you can pivot lightly on this last down-step so that you will be Scooting back at a slightly different angle.

Now Scoot back to the left on the next 8 beats, rising on LF, pulling in your RF, keeping your weight on your RF and leaning to right. Again, step down strongly on 7 and transfer your weight to LF. Hold the next beat.

From here, exit the Scoots, for example by easing back into the second half of the Basic or switching into Out and Ins.

You don't need to Scoot for exactly 8 counts if you don't feel like it or if you do not have enough side space, but the count needs to be an even number. You can keep the "Scoots" shorter, and even ease back into the Balboa Basic right after the first two side steps.

Paddles and Snakes

Paddles are similar to Scoots, but while Scoots move in a straight line sideways, Paddles are circular, moving either clockwise or counter-clockwise.

You could say that Paddles are Scoots done in a circle. For this reason, Paddles are sometimes also referred to as Balboa Circles.

Paddling counter-clockwise

From the Balboa Basic, step down firmly on 3, lean into it, hold on 4, and then "Paddle" counter-clockwise, turning continuously to left (8 single counts). Always step forward on right foot, going up on the ball of your foot, while your left foot stays down flat and turns more or less on one spot, bearing your weight. You pretty much Paddle around your left foot as an anchor.

The follower will mirror what you do. She will Paddle around her right foot which is placed close to your left foot, forming a common axis. She will step back on LF when you step forward on RF.

After 8 beats, continue Paddling counter-clockwise but change your footwork for variety.

On 7, step down firmly on RF and transfer your weight to it. On 8, swing your LF by and behind your RF without stepping down, pivot a quarter to left and then step down on 1 on LF.

From here, continue Paddling still counter-clockwise but now backwards, stepping down on LF on 3, 5 and 7, and pulling in your RF on 2, 4 and 6. Step down firmly on 7, pivot slightly to right, switch back to the original footwork and Paddle 8 more counts counter-clockwise, finally easing back into a Balboa Basic.

Paddling back and forth

Instead of Paddling continuously counter-clockwise, you can reverse direction after the first 8 beats and Paddle back to where you came from.

On 7, step down firmly on RF, transfer your weight to it and hold on 8. Then Paddle back, this time turning continuously to right, stepping on LF on 1, 3, 5 and 7, while your right foot stays down flat and turns more or less on one spot, bearing your weight.

At the end, ease back into the Balboa Basic.

The Snake

Pivot a quarter to right when you step down on 7, then on the next 8 beats continue Paddling forward, but now moving to your left. Do 8 beats to right and 8 beats to left, the turns connected with a strong down-step and hold.

This figure, Paddling alternatingly to left and to right but aiming forward throughout, is called "Snakes" or "Serpentine". It looks as if you are winding your way forward in an S-shape like a snake. The rhythm is: "1-2-3-4-5-6-7-hold", repeat.

You can alternate the direction more frequently if you wish, for example pivoting on 3 or 5 (instead of 7).

You can also do the Snake backwards if there is enough space behind you (although I am not sure whether snakes can move in this fashion).

Come Around

The Come Around is a variation of the Basic Step and an important, frequently used figure of Balboa.

It is a circular 8-count figure, where you both turn to the right on 3 and "come around" each other (or change places), doing a roughly 180 turn by the end of the 8 beats.

Stay in closed position and do not separate during this figure.

The first 4 beats are danced "down", and the second 4 beats are danced "up" like this:
- Step-step-step-hold
- Step-step-hold-step

On 3, step down firmly on LF, somewhat forward and diagonally to left, while starting to turn to right. Lead the follower to do the same. Hold on 4, but keep pivoting to right on LF.

On 5, continue turning to right and step on RF behind and across your LF.

On 6, close your LF to your RF.

Hold on 7, then step back on 8. You have now made an approximately 180 turn around the imaginary axis between the two of you.

Promenade

"Promenade" refers to a dance position that is also commonly used in many other dances.

Promenade position (PP) is a "semi-open" position where the leader, standing with the follower in closed position, turns slightly to his left and the follower turns slightly to her right. As a result, his right shoulder touches her left shoulder, their other shoulder moves away from each other, and their upper bodies form a slight V-shape, open to the leader's left. His feet and head also turns to left, and hers to right.

In this way, the couple opens up the closed position on one side, namely the side of the handhold, usually in preparation for a move sideways to the leader's left, although it is possible to get into a Promenade and then get out of it right away without taking any steps to the side.

In Balboa, there are many ways to get into Promenade position. You can, for example, do a Come Around, open it up into Promenade position on 5-6, and step forward on 7. Hold on 8.

Or you can do the following popular 8-count figure to get into PP:

Dance the first half of the Balboa Basic. On 5, step to side to your right on RF. On 6, turn to left into Promenade position and step forward on LF (i.e. step to left relative to your original direction). Step forward an 7, flex your knee, and hold on 8. The follower will mirror your steps 5 to 8.

Lolly Kicks

Lolly Kicks, also called Lollie Kicks or Lollies, can be described as assuming Promenade position and rhythmically turning toward and away from each other. When turning toward each other, you both tap down with the ball of your outside foot, and when turning away into PP, you both kick forward with your inside foot.

You can get into the Lollies, for example, from a Come Around. Do a Come Around but on 7, open her up into Promenade position and you both kick forward with your inside (your right, her left) foot. On 8, turn against each other and step down.

From here, turn towards each other and tap down on 1, kick forward on 3, tap down on 5, kick forward on 7 and so on. Between the taps and kicks, on the even beats, step down with your kicking/tapping foot and turn to the direction of the next kick or tap.

When you tap down, compress your hands. When you kick forward, get a stretch from your handhold. These compressions and stretches are repeated during the Lollies. Stretch, compress, stretch, compress. Keep your left hand halfway between the two of you in a steady position, and do not start moving it back and forth as if sawing on a log.

The "kick" is not really a kick in the air. It comes more from the hip, brushing the floor and swinging out your foot.

You can also get into Lollies from the Balboa Basic or right from standing in closed position. Simply start turning towards and away from the follower to the rhythm of the Lollies, leading her to do the same, and then launch into the taps and kicks. This can also be a good way to start a dance.

You can learn to add various turns (hers and/or yours) to the Lollies, explained later in the bonus steps section.

You can exit the Lollies in many ways, for example by switching into Out and Ins, going into a Come Around or a Toss-Out, or doing a Pop Turn.

Pop Turn

A Pop Turn occurs when the follower is on your right side and you "pop" her into a free left turn toward you.

A "free turn" is when the person turning has no hand contact with his or her partner while turning.

The side-by-side position is similar to that during the Lollies, and you can get into this position just like you did with the Lollies, for example from a Come Around. Do a Come Around, but on 7 open her up into a side-by-side position (she is on your right) and kick forward with your inside foot. Keep your right hand on her back.

This time turn her out even more on 7 in order to compress your right hand and your lower arm on her back to build momentum for her turn. Now step down on 8 and lead her into a free turn to left. You lead her turn with your left hand only.

You can choose whether to lead the follower to do her free spin to your right (behind you) or to your left (in front of you). You do this with the angle and pressure of your arm, and the movement of your body.

Led to your right

If you want to lead her to spin toward your right (or aiming behind you from the starting side-by-side position), then step forward and turn to right to get out of her way as she spins, then continue turning to right, make a U-turn, and position yourself to pick her up face-to-face in closed dance position at the end of her turn. Your footwork while making this U-turn is "1-2-3-hold".

Led to your left

If you want to lead her to spin to your left (or aiming in front of you from the starting side-by-side position) then step back and turn to left to get out of her way as she spins, then continue turning left, follow her as she spins, and position yourself to pick her up face-to-face in closed dance position at the end of her turn. You can then use the momentum of her turn to continue into Pivot Turns to left after you pick her up.

Notice a significant difference between leading the follower's free turn to your right versus to your left. Turning to your right is only a half turn for the follower, but turning to your left is a turn and a half for her, so she has to spin more and faster.

Pivot Turns

The Pivot Turn is a turn that the leader and follower do moving together in closed position. It can be danced turning to right or turning to left. It is done in "slow" even steps, stepping down on every second beat and turning continuously.

To dance the Pivot Turn to right, start with doing the first half of a Come Around. As you step down on 3 (LF), already turning to right, continue that right turn by stepping on the odd beats: 5 (RF), 7 (LF) etc. Always step forward on left foot, and then close your right foot, pivoting to right on each step. Continue the Pivot Turns for as long as you wish.

When you want to exit, wait for the next step down on LF and continue into the second half of the Come Around.

Alternatively, after stepping down on RF, stop the rotation and switch to Out-and-Ins.

Or, after a step forward on LF, step to side on RF sliding out a little to the side and then hold for a beat. Your left foot is now free to start any new figure.

To dance the Pivot Turn to left, do an Out and In. As you step down on 7 (RF), make that a longer step and start turning to left. Continue the left turn stepping down on the odd beats: 1 (LF), 3 (RF) etc. Always step forward on right foot, and then close your left foot, pivoting to left throughout.

To exit, step to side on 7 (RF), sliding out a little to the side and hold for one beat (7-&). Your left foot is now free to start any step.

The Pivot Turn is a versatile step and can be added to many figures.

The axis of the Pivot Turns is between the two of you, and you use each other's weight as the momentum for the continuing turns.

Doing 4 steps (8 beats) are generally enough, but you can continue the Pivot Turn longer if you want, just don't get dizzy.

Underarm Turn

This figure is an inside (left) underarm turn of the follower. Similar figures are known in other swing dances and may be called "Change of Places". You will dance it "down", i.e. stepping down on 3 and 7.

Dance a Balboa Basic Box. When you start the next Basic, do a rock step on 1-2 leading the follower to also do a rock step, mirroring you. Step forward and diagonally left on 3, turning slightly to right and lifting your left hand up and across your chest to lead an Underarm Turn (inside left turn). She will start turning and moving in front of you from left to right. On 4, hold your foot but continue turning her. At this point she is showing you her back, having already started her turn.

As she continues turning, step forward and turn to right to follow her and be in front of her as she completes her turn (1-2-&-4). Pick her up and continue dancing.

You can double the fun by making this into a Double Underarm Turn. Keep your hand up after her first turn to signal that she is to make another turn, and bring it down only at the end of her second turn to signal that she should stop turning. Since it takes two more beats and steps for the follower to make a second turn, you will also need to add two more single steps ("step-step") while she turns.

Similarly, you can make this into a triple turn. Add yet two more single steps ("step-step-step-step") while she turns. Use these steps to follow her as she turns and position yourself to be in front of her when she is done turning.

Keep your hand above her head and lead the turns with small circular movements of your hand. If you make too wide circles with your hand, she may lose her balance.

When the follower makes two or more turns in a row, she does not always end up where you expect her to end up, so be flexible, make sure to follow her and be in position to pick her up at the end.

Note that if the follower turns the other way (outside or right underarm turn) that is called a Tuck Turn (described later).

Toss-Out with Free Turn

The Toss-Out, also called "Throw-Out" or "Bal Swingout", is a signature Balboa move. It inserts 8 more beats between the first 4 beats and the last 4 beats of the Come Around, for a total of 16 beats. The 8 extra beats consist of a stretch and then an inside turn (left turn) of the follower.

Dance the first 4 beats of the Come Around. On 5-6, continue turning to right but release your right arm from the follower's back, separate from her and get into a face-to-face open position, the left-to-right handhold now extended toward each other. This separation and letting her step away is the "toss-out" or "throw-out" part of the figure. From here, numerous alternative resolutions could follow, the most common being the follower's inside free turn.

The follower's free turn is a stretch turn, meaning that the momentum comes from a stretch of the arms as the leader and follower step away from each other.

Just as with the Pop Turn, you can choose whether to lead the follower's inside free spin to you right or to your left.

Led to your right

Leading it to your right is the common way and it goes like this:

On 7, you both lean back a little, kick forward and give each other a good stretch which will wind her up for her turn. On 8, step down and lead her into a free inside spin in front of you, moving from your left to your right.

Let go of her hand, step forward as she turns and make a U-turn to the right to position yourself to be in front of her when she completes her spin. Skim her waist with the fingers of your right hand as she turns, let your hand come to rest on her back and pick her up in closed position (1-2-3-hold). From here, complete the last 4 beats of the Come Around.

The footwork of the 16 beats will be:

- First 4 beats: Step-step-down-& (first half of the Come Around)

- Mid 8 beats: Step-step-kick-step-<u>step-step</u>-down-& (Toss-Out and Free Turn)
- Last 4 beats: Step-step-hold-step (second half of the Come Around)

The two underlined steps are when the follower does her free turn.

During her turn, she should keep her left hand up, to be ready to put it back on your shoulder. This is a principle of following, to keep her hand at approximately the same level where it was when contact was lost, so that contact can be re-established smoothly.

However, she should also avoid hitting you in the face or chest with her elbow while she turns, ideally. This is commonly accomplished by her making a "brushing her hair" move with her left hand just before you pick her up.

Led to your left

If you want to lead the follower's free spin to your left, then turn less than usual on 5-6 and do not face her on 7. Instead, show her your right shoulder and reach across your chest with your left hand to hold her right hand and give her that stretch.

On 7, you both kick forward and give each other a good stretch which will wind her up for a turn. On 8, step down and lead her into a free inside spin in front of you from your right to your left.

Now step forward and make a U-turn to left to be in front of her when she completes her spin, place your right hand on her back and pick her up in closed position (1-2-3-hold).

Note that while leading the free turn to your right is a comfortable half turn for the follower, leading it to your left is a turn and a half for her, so she has to spin more and faster.

Toss-Out with Underarm Turn

The Toss-Out with Underarm Turn is practically identical to the Toss-Out with Free Turn except you will now lead an underarm turn instead of a free turn.

The direction of follower's rotation will be the same as previously, but this time do not let go of her hand on beat 8. Instead, raise your left hand and lead an Underarm Turn.

The timing of raising and lowering your left hand is important. Make sure to lift your hand in time to signal the coming Underarm Turn, and bring it down at the end of her turn to stop the turning motion. This, and your right hand on her back will signal to her that the turn is over and she should not continue turning.

Behind-the-Back Toss-Out

While the follower does her turn during a Toss-Out with Free Turn, the leader normally keeps facing her and only turns enough to follow her and step into her when she has completed her turn.

To add more spice to this figure, you can also do a free left turn of your own while the follower turns. You will not hold her hand while you turn, so the turn will be a free turn for both of you.

Because of your added turn, the preparation for this figure will look somewhat like a Toss-Out with Free Turn led to your left, even though the follower's turn is led to your right as in the common Toss-Out variant. You just have to position yourself differently

On 5-6 of the Toss-Out, turn less than usual and do not face the follower on 7. Instead, show her your right shoulder and reach across your chest with your left hand to hold her right hand and give her that stretch.

On 7, you both kick forward as usual and give each other a good stretch. This will now serve to wind up both of you for a turn. On 8, step down and lead her into a free inside spin behind your back. Let go of her hand and while she turns do a half turn to left yourself, moving towards her.

Note that whether you add a left turn or not, you will have to follow approximately the same path on the floor in order to be in front of her when she completes her turn.

In effect, both of you will make an approximately 180 turn while passing by each other and trading places. At the end of your turn, reach out with your right hand to catch her, place your hand on her back and pick her up in closed position. From here, complete the last 4 beats of the Come Around.

Start your own turn already on 8. Depending on your relative heights, let go of her hand over your right shoulder (if she is tall), or outside your right arm, or at waist level (if she is short). Even though you are also turning, try to keep an eye on the follower as much as possible and make sure to be in front of her when she completes her spin. This can be challenging because you have to correctly position yourself while you turn.

As you see, the Toss-Out can indeed serve as the base for a variety of turns.

Bonus Balboa figures

This chapter introduces a few more Balboa figures that can help make your dancing richer and more enjoyable.

<u>Swivels</u>

To dance the Swivels, first you need to get into Promenade position (PP). Do this using one of the ways described previously.

You are now standing with the follower on your right side in Promenade position, your weight on your RF forward and her weight on her LF forward.

The Swivels are done with the dancers facing each other in closed position, standing about one foot apart, and moving sideways on a line or slot alternatingly to the left and to the right. The leader's basic footwork is as follows:

1. From PP, step forward on LF and pivot to right to face the follower
2. Small step back on RF
3. Step sideways to right on LF, crossing in front of RF
4. Hold on 4
5. Step sideways to right on RF, crossing behind LF
6. Small step back on LF
7. Step sideways to left, RF crossing in front of LF
8. Hold on 8

The follower will mirror your steps throughout.

This is the basic footwork to which you will add the actual "swivels" at each step.

"Swivel" means a twisting motion of the lower body where the hips and the legs pivot from side to side on the balls of the feet, but the upper body (torso) and arms remains relatively motionless.

You will swivel to Right (1), Left (2), Right (3), and then to Left (5), Right (6), Left (7). "Swivel-Swivel-Cross, Swivel-Swivel-Cross". The follower will mirror you, and you will both leverage on each other to give momentum to each swivel.

Typically during the Swivels, the follower will do most of the swiveling and her swivels will be more pronounced than yours. It is really her chance to shine, and you do not need to swivel too much.

Exit the Swivels after "7-&" by doing a rock step and continuing into a Come Around.

Toss-Out with Double Free Turn

Once you get comfortable with the basic Toss-Out and its various add-on turns, you can try doubling and varying those turns.

Start with the basic Toss-Out with Free Turn led to your right, and add a second Free Turn of the follower immediately after her first turn.

As far as leading this second turn is concerned, it does not actually require any particular leading. If you do not catch the follower after her first turn, she should just continue turning. This is a principle of following, to continue repeating a move if the leader does not stop or change the movement.

As you recall, your footwork for the Toss-Out with a single Free Turn was:
Step-step-kick-step-<u>step-step</u>-down-&
(the steps when the follower does her free turn are underlined)

Because a second turn will take two steps for the follower to complete, you will also need to add two more single steps in order to lead a double free turn, so the figure will require a total of 18 beats instead of 16.

Your footwork for the Toss-Out and two free turns of the follower will be:
Step-step-kick-step-<u>step-step-step-step</u>-down-&
(the steps when she does her two turns are underlined)

In other words, just do another "step-step" while she continues into the second spin, following her as necessary, then catch her at the end of the second spin the same way you did in the original, single turn version.

Note that a "single turn" is actually only a half turn for the follower, but a "double turn" is a turn and a half for her, so she has to spin more and faster.

Toss-Out with Double Underarm Turn

You can also double the follower's Underarm Turn after a Toss-Out. Here too, take two more single steps and use it to lead another underarm turn immediately after the first.

Your footwork for the Toss-Out and two underarm turns of the follower will be:
Step-step-kick-step-<u>step-step-step-step</u>-down-&
(the steps when she does her two turns are underlined)

The timing of raising and lowering your left hand is important.

Lift your hand in time to signal the coming underarm turn to the follower, keep it up to signal that she is to continue turning and make another turn, and bring it down only at the end of her second turn to signal that she should not turn any more.

Note that, while the follower's single turn is actually only a half turn, the "double turn" is a turn and a half for her, so she has to turn more and faster.

Toss-Out with Underarm Turn and Free Turn

Instead of leading the same type of turn twice, you can lead an Underarm Turn first, followed immediately by a Free Turn.

The timing of raising and lowering your left hand is important. Make sure to lift your hand in time to signal the coming Underarm Turn to the follower. Bring your hand down at the end of her first turn, but do not stop her turning motion. Instead, continue leading a Free Turn and let go of her hand at waist level to allow her to continue spinning freely.

Pick her up at the end of her Free Turn the same way you did with a single Free Turn: by putting your right hand on her back and catching her right hand with your left hand, to signal that the turn is over and she should not continue turning.

This again is an 18-beat figure in total.

Your footwork for the Toss-Out and the two turns is the same as with the previous double turns:
Step-step-kick-step-step-step-step-step-down-&
(the steps when she does her two turns are underlined)

She will do an Underarm Turn during the first "step-step" and a Free Turn during the second "step-step".

Toss-Out and Pop Turn combinations

When you have completed a Toss-Out with one of the turns and picked up the follower in closed position, you will usually dance the second half of the Come Around to conclude the figure.

But you can also choose to transform that second half of the Come Around into a new Toss-Out with another type of turn. For example, if the turn of your first Toss-Out was a Free Turn, then lead an Underarm Turn. You may then continue immediately into a third Toss-Out and lead a Behind-the-Back.

Another option is to add further variety by transforming the second half of the Come Around into a Pop Turn.

With Free Turns, Underarm Turns, Behind-the-Backs, Pop Turns, single, double or triple turns, and turns led to you right or to your left, the possibilities are almost endless.

Texas Tommy

This figure is also popular in other swing dances where it may go under various names such as "Handshake behind the Back" or "Apache Turn".

In essence, the figure consists of passing the follower's right hand behind her back from your left hand to you right hand, and then leading a follower's turn to "untangle" this behind-the-back handhold position. Lastly, you will need to lead an additional free turn to switch the resulting R2R ("handshake") handhold back to the regular L2R handhold.

The Texas Tommy is often added to the Toss-Out with Underarm Turn. This adds 8 more beats or counts to the already 16-count figure, for a total of 24 counts. Breaking it down to its components, the sequence looks like this:

- 1/ First half of the Come Around   (4 beats)
- 2/ Toss-Out and stretch   (4 beats)
- 3/ Follower's Underarm Turn   (4 beats)
- 4/ Follower's right turn with Texas Tommy   (4 beats)
- 5/ Follower's left Free Turn   (4 beats)

47

- 6/ Second half of the Come Around (4 beats)

The Texas Tommy starts at the end of part 3/ when you make a U-turn to the right to pick up the follower after her Underarm Turn (1-2-3-&). On 3-&, your right hand should already be on her back and your left hand should be catching her right hand.

With a smooth continuation of this motion, gently reach around her with your left hand, moving her right hand behind her back at waist level. Place her hand, palm out, on her lower back and pass it to your right hand. It is generally easier to take her wrist with your right hand and then let her hand slide into yours. Keep your hands low and your arms relaxed. You are now in a right-to-right ("handshake") handhold, albeit behind her back.

On 1-2-3 of part 4/ of the sequence, you will use your right hand to lead the follower into a right turn to "untangle" the handhold. Move out of her way as she steps forward to turn, but do not release the R2R handhold while she turns. Keep the handhold loose and do not grip her hand, so that it can turn in yours. Your hands will stretch at the end of her turn.

In part 5/ of the sequence, use the momentum of that stretch to lead her back into a free left turn with your right hand. Release her hand at this point. From here, the figure is like a Toss-Out with Free Turn and you can complete it accordingly.

The follower's three consecutive turns (left-right-left) in parts 3/ to 5/ of the sequence come back-to-back, immediately one after the other, so she will have a lot of turning to do in those 12 counts.

It is very important to keep the follower's hand low, at the level of her waist and lower back. Keep your hands low and relaxed to avoid straining her arm. The follower must also keep her right arm loose and relaxed for the Texas Tommy to work. Never force the Texas Tommy as it can lead to injuries.

The Texas Tommy is a great-looking move and it can be added as a variation to other steps as well.

Beach Pushes

The name of this figure is a reference to the famous black & white video clip showing young couples dancing Balboa and Collegiate Shag in a beachside parking lot at Venice Beach, California in 1938. One of the couples is seen performing the "Beach Pushes".

Similar figures are also used in other dances and are variously known as "Pancake" or "Hand to Hand".

Beach Pushes essentially look like this: The partners are separated, standing face-to-face about one step apart, and they turn repeatedly to their respective left and right (i.e. into opposite directions relative to each other). When they turn to their left, their extended right hands meet and their palms compress (push) against each other in cross-handhold. When they turn to their right, their left hands meet and compress.

The momentum of the compressions stops the turn to one direction and initiates the turn into the opposite direction.

Not only the handhold changes from the usual "left-to-right" to "cross-handhold", but the basic footwork of the dancers relative to each other changes as well.

Normally you and the follower step on opposite foot, i.e. when you step on LF she steps on RF and vice versa. Only this way can you step together in closed position.

But to do the Beach Pushes, you and the follower will need to step on the same foot: both of you on LF at the same time, and both of you on RF at the same time. This is possible to do because you are now separated from each other.

To get into this type of footwork, one of you will have to switch footwork and align it with the other's by taking one more or one less step than the other.

As you will see, it will be you who takes one less step than the follower when you get into the Beach Pushes. You will then again take one step less when you exit the figure, in order to switch your footwork back to normal at the end.

To enter the Beach Pushes

Since the handhold differs from the usual, a good opportunity to get into the Beach Pushes comes after a free turn when hand contact is released and a new handhold can be assumed at the end of the turn.

For example, do a Toss-Out with Free Turn led to your right, but this time after 7-8, do not step forward and turn to right to pick up the follower after her Free Turn.

Instead, on the next 4 beats take two slow steps while she does her turn:

1. Step to side on LF
2. Hold
3. Turn a quarter to left, step forward on RF and extend your right hand to your side to meet her right hand when she completes her turn
4. Hold

You took 2 steps and she took 3 steps, so you are now on the same foot (RF), roughly side by side, facing the opposite direction, palms of your right hands touching and compressing.

She does not need to worry about changing her footwork, in fact she should not even notice that you changed yours if you do it smoothly.

It is of course possible to get into the Beach Pushes from many other figures. If a free turn is not involved, then you will need to simply and smoothly change the handhold from L2R to R2R.

To do the Beach Pushes

From this position, do the Beach Pushes, alternatingly turning left and right. Your footwork is:

1. Step forward on LF and pivot 180 to right
2. Step forward on RF
3. Step forward on LF and compress hands
4. Hold
5. Step forward on RF and pivot 180 to left
6. Step forward on LF
7. Step forward on RF and compress hands
8. Hold

Repeat. Use the compression of the palms (the "pushes") to give momentum to your pivots into the opposite direction. Do not stay too close to each other and remember to pulse.

To exit the Beach Pushes

To exit, use the next left-to-left handhold to lead the follower into a free left turn. While she turns, you will have to switch your footwork again as follows.

You are on your LF, facing to your right with your extended left hand meeting her extended left hand.

5. Step forward on RF and turn 180 to left

6. Hold
7. Step forward on LF, turning after her if necessary, preparing to pick her up
8. Hold your foot and pick her up

You took 2 steps while she took 3 steps, so you are now "back to normal".

From here, proceed the same way as you would with completing a Toss-Out with Free Turn, i.e. dance the second half of the Basic.

As always, there are many other ways to get out of the Beach Pushes.

Reverse Toss-Out with Free Turn

"Reverse" refers to the fact that in this version of the Toss-Out the follower will separate to your right (not to your left), and you will lead her turn with your right hand (not with your left).

Dance a Come Around, but on 7 open her up into a side-by-side position (she is on your right). This is similar to the Lollies, but this time do not keep your right hand on her back. Instead, let your hand slide down on her arm and catch her right hand as she separates and steps away from you. This way you are "tossing her out" to your right. Your handhold is now right-to-left.

On 7, you both kick forward and give each other a good stretch which will wind her up for her turn. From here, various alternatives could follow, the most common being the follower's inside (left) free turn.

Just as with the Pop Turn, you can choose whether to lead the follower's free turn to you right or to your left.

She will turn to left in either case, but as she steps forward to turn, she can aim in front of you or behind you, as you stand side-by-side, depending on your lead.

Led to your right

If you lead her to spin to your right (aiming behind you as you stand side-by-side), then step forward and turn to right to get out of her way as she spins, then continue turning to right and position yourself so that you can pick her up face-to-face in closed dance position at the end of her turn. Your footwork is "1-2-3-hold".

Led to your left

If you lead her to spin to your left (aiming in front of you as you stand side-by-side), then step back and turn to left to get out of her way as she spins, then continue turning left following her, and position yourself so that you can pick her up face-to-face in closed dance position at the end of her turn.

Since you are now both turning left, you can use that momentum to continue into Pivot Turns to left.

Note that leading the free turn to your right is a half turn for the follower, but leading it to your left is a turn and a half for her.

<u>Tuck Turn</u>

The Tuck Turn is a common figure is most swing dances. It is an outside (right) underarm turn of the follower.

The Tuck Turn is a compression turn, meaning that the momentum for the turn comes from the hands of the leader and follower pressing against each other.

Here the Tuck Turn is done in 8 counts with Balboa footwork. The figure is danced "up" like this:

- step-step-hold-step
- step-step-kick-step

Dance the first 4 beats of a Balboa Basic, but on 3 pull back your left shoulder and lift your left knee. This will turn her slightly to her left and wind her up for the coming Tuck Turn. Step down on 4 and start leading a follower's underarm right turn (outside turn).

You can give more momentum to the winding-up by leading a rock step on 1, and then turning her out to her right on 2, before dancing 3-4 as described above.

Continue leading an underarm outside turn on 5-6. When she completed her turn, you have several options to proceed.

You can, for example, stay in face-to-face open position after her turn (5-6). Bring your hand down on 6 and kick to the left with your right foot on 7, giving her a stretch. Step down on 8. Continue into a Toss-Out with a turn of your choice as follows.

Tuck Turn and Toss-Out

One option would be to use the Tuck Turn as a replacement for the Toss-Out and to immediately lead another turn after the Tuck Turn, just as you would after the Toss-Out.

This is because at beat 7 of the Tuck Turn you are in the same position as at beat 7 of the Toss-Out. You just arrived here differently, replacing the Come Around with a Tuck Turn.

You can therefore easily continue the Tuck Turn with leading a Free Turn of the follower. Do this exactly as described under the figure Toss-Out with Free Turn.

The Free Turn is of course not the only thing you can lead after the Tuck Turn. You can lead an Underarm Turn, a Behind-the-Back, Texas Tommy or any other turn, double turn, triple turn or combination of turns as you would after the Toss-Out.

Tuck Turn with Elbow Catch

At the end of the Tuck Turn, on 7, instead of the usual kick to the left and stretch, step down firmly on right foot and (gently) grab the follower's right elbow, upper arm or shoulder to stop her turn, and then spin her back into the opposite direction.

You can use your right hand or your left hand to grab her right elbow. It does not matter which hand you use.

If you use your right hand, then you will need to reach across to catch her right arm as she turns.

It is somewhat easier to use your left hand because it is closer to her right arm and does not require reaching across.

Lollies with Turns

You can make the Lolly Kicks more interesting by inserting turns for the follower, and even a free turn of your own.

During the Lollies, lead the follower into outside (right) or inside (left) free turns as follows.

Leading an outside (right) free turn of the follower

The follower's outside turn is a compression turn, meaning that the momentum comes from the hands of the leader and follower pressing against each other.

Do a couple of Lolly Kicks. When it comes to a "tap", step down firmly on your outside foot (1/ LF) and compress your hand firmly against the follower's hand. This indicates to her that a right turn is coming. Hold on the next beat (2), then lead an outside free turn on the following two beats (3-4). To accommodate the follower's free turn, which takes two beats to complete, add to your footwork two single steps in-place while she turns (RF-LF). At the end of her turn, pick her up and continue leading the Lollies with a "kick" (RF).

Therefore, instead of the usual "tap-turn-kick-turn", your footwork will be "step-hold-step-step-kick-turn". The two beats where her turn takes place are underlined.

If you want to lead a double outside turn, then just increase the intensity of the compression slightly, do not pick her up after her first turn, and add yet two more single steps to your footwork: "step-hold-step-step-step-step-kick-turn".

Again, you do not need to actually "lead" the second turn. If you do not catch the follower after her first turn, she should just continue turning.

Leading an inside (left) free turn of the follower

This will be an easy figure if you are already familiar with the Toss-Out.

In contrast to the outside turn which is a compression turn, the inside turn is a stretch turn, meaning that the momentum comes from a stretch of the arms as the leader and follower step away from each other.

During the Lollies, after a "tap" with your left foot (1), step back on LF (2), away from the follower to create some distance between you. Now lean back slightly and kick forward and down with right foot, creating a stretch (3). Step down on RF and use the momentum of the stretch to lead an inside free turn (4).

It takes two steps for the follower to complete her turn. You will therefore need to also take two steps in place (LF-RF). As she completes her turn, put your right hand on her back, catch her right hand and continue leading the Lollies with a tap (LF). Your footwork is: "tap-step-kick-step-<u>step-step</u>-tap-turn".

As you can see, this move is very similar to 7-8 of the Toss-Out, except this time you do not step in a U-turn after the follower as she completes her turn. Rather, you stay in place and continue leading the Lollies after her turn.

If you want to lead a double inside free turn from the Lollies, then just let her do a second turn before picking her up, and add yet two more single steps to your footwork: "tap-step-kick-step-<u>step-step-step-step</u>-tap-turn".

The similarity to the Toss-Out also suggests a possible exit from the Lollies. Lead a follower's inside free turn from the Lollies, and turn it into a Toss-Out with Free Turn, i.e. step after her turning right in a U-shape while she spins, pick her up in closed position and dance the second half of the Come Around.

Leading underarm turns (instead of free turns)

It is probably needless to say at this point that you can also lead underarm turns instead of free turns from the Lollies, if you wish. This applies to both the inside and outside turns, both single or double.

The outside turn will be a Tuck Turn, and the inside turn will be an Underarm Turn.

Refer to previous comments concerning single and double underarm turns, in particular regarding the timing of raising and lowering your left hand.

Leader's right turn

When you lead an inside (left) free turn of the follower, as described above, you can simultaneously perform a free right turn of your own. This full turn takes two steps to complete and replaces the two steps-in-place that you would otherwise do.

Simultaneous turns of the follower and the leader always look great if done properly.

Normally you would use the stretch to give momentum only to her turn. This time, use the stretch to give momentum to each of you to do you respective turns.

You can watch this relatively simple figure beautifully presented in the short Balboa dance scene in the 1938 Hollywood movie "Start Cheering".

The Slide

The Slide is a simple and elegant move. It can be used to temporarily slow down the dance, and to break the basic rhythm and the constant rotations with a side move.

Dance a Come-Around, except on 5 slide your right foot out sideways to the right, transferring your weight fully to it. Then pull in your left foot slowly and gradually over 6-7-8.

In keeping with the generally limited footprint of Balboa, the extent of the side slide does not need to be long.

This move can be done at any time during a song, but it is especially effective when used to end a dance.

Maxie's Stop and Slide

"Maxie's Stop and Slide" is a short choreography named after Maxie Dorf, a well-known Balboa dancer who was active in the 1930s and 40s and has contributed greatly to the more recent revival of the dance.

Dance a couple of Lollies, then change the "kicks and taps" into four quick swivels-in-place in double tempo (QQQQ), then drop your weight (Q) and slide out both of your feet to the side (Q). Keep your head level during the slide-out.

This is the "Stop" part of the figure.

The "Maxie Slide" consists of a "ball-change", followed by a Slide to right.

As you stand with your feet apart, take a small step back on the ball of your RF ("ball"/Q), step across to right with your LF in front of your RF, with your knee bent ("change"/Q), and take a wide step/slide to right on RF transferring your weight fully to your RF. Pull in your left foot to your RF slowly and gradually.

During the slide, look back to left and leave your trailing left shoulder down.

Social dancing

When you have already learned and practiced the various steps and figures of Balboa, the next level in your Balboa journey is to become a competent social dancer.

The rest of this book contains some observations on practicing, leading, following and social dancing.

Going to a swing social dance generally should not be an intimidating experience even for a beginner. The music is lively and happy and people tend to be friendly.

There may be groups of experienced dancers or instructors who know each other and may keep to themselves in one area, or groups of friends who prefer to dance with each other, but generally speaking you may dance with most anyone.

Type of the social dance event

If you are lucky, you may be able to find local dance parties specifically for Balboa, often hosted by Balboa clubs. These will feature fast swing music suitable for dancing Balboa.

If Balboa parties are not available, the next best opportunities will be offered by more general swing dance parties, where the tempo of the music will likely vary from slow to fast.

A swing dance event will generally tend toward a particular type of swing dance, based on the organizers' preferences. In most cases this will be either Lindy Hop, or East Coast Swing/Jive, or West Coast Swing. For a student of Balboa, a Lindy Hop dance party is the best option, although East Coast Swing events, which tend to play more of the 1950s rock and roll music, may also be suitable for dancing Balboa.

West Coast Swing, however is a significantly different dance, and one will not be able to dance Balboa to the music played there.

Recurring social dances are typically organized by dance schools, swing dance or swing music organizations, or dance halls and other venues that host all kinds of events. Information on these events as well as upcoming classes and special workshops is generally readily available online.

When you choose a social dance to attend, it is worth paying attention to who the DJ will be, or whether a live band will be playing, because often a particular DJ or band tends to play a certain kind of music, and some may be more to your liking than others.

Tempo of the music

At the more general swing (usually Lindy Hop) dance parties the tempo of the music will vary widely. At events like this, the tempo of the music can actually become an issue.

The issue is that if you only know how to dance Balboa, then you will sit a lot and watch others dance to slower music. For this reason, it is a good idea to learn at least one more swing dance that you can dance to mid-tempo music. It is also more fun to enjoy various dances than to dance only Balboa all the time.

Dancers who only know one swing dance will often try to force that particular dance to a tempo that it is not suited for. This is generally a losing battle. It is a much better approach to pick an appropriate dance to the given tempo of music.

Swing dancing has many varieties and each variety is naturally suited to a certain tempo of music. The following are some of these dances (with the optimal range of tempo in beats per minute indicated in brackets) from very slow to very fast:

> Blues (40-80 BPM) → Slow Balboa; slower variants of Foxtrot (80-120) → Lindy Hop (120-160) → Lindy Hop with Charleston footwork; Jive and East Coast Swing (140-180) → Single-time Jive/ECS (160-200) → Classic Charleston and Break-away; Balboa (180-220) → Ragtime One-Step

During a swing social dance, if the music is pleasant mid-tempo, you will probably want to dance Lindy Hop, which is the most versatile swing dance.

Faster music generally requires that you keep your steps smaller and tighter, your partner closer, your pulsing shallower, and cut out any "unnecessary" body movements (like triple steps) where possible. The swing dances which have these characteristics and therefore suit fast music better are the Charleston, the Break-Away and the Balboa.

Dancing to slow swing music can be even more challenging than dancing to fast or mid-tempo music. Slow dancing generally requires increased smoothness and fluidity of movement, and completing each movement to the fullest. Slow Foxtrot is a sophisticated and elegant ballroom dance, but it is difficult to learn. It is also a progressive or travelling dance that may be impossible to do when everyone else is doing spot dances (i.e. dancing in one spot). Blues is also a slow dance but due to its overtly sensual nature it is mostly danced at Blues events and not well suited to a general swing dance party.

It is probably fair to say that the best spot dance for slow swing music is the elegant and easy to learn Slow Balboa.

Variety and playfulness

Although at first every dance seems complicated and difficult to the beginner, once it is mastered it becomes increasingly simple to do, and with this, the danger arises that it also becomes increasingly repetitive and boring.

To keep Balboa from becoming boring, use a good mix of figures that vary in type, footwork, complexity and direction of body movement, but always in harmony with the music.

Simple things like changing the dance hold and the distance between the partners, dancing once in close embrace and then opening up a little, even when doing the same figure, or holding your left hand sometimes slightly higher and sometimes slightly lower, add to variety.

Don't be too stiff in your dance hold. Balboa is a happy dance, so feel free to express the happy feeling it generates. Keep your upper body flexible and allow it to move and tilt in different directions as the momentum of the figures inspires it.

Generally, the less uptight one feels toward a dance, and the more one makes the dance his own, the more opportunities open up to make it interesting.

Try to improvise by taking apart the figures you know, breaking them down to their components and putting the parts together differently, so that somehow it still makes sense in reflection to the music.

To successfully improvise a dance, one will of course need a good follower who is quick, flexible and able to react instantaneously.

Starting and ending a dance

It is more fun to make the beginning and the end of a dance more interesting than simply just starting and stopping to dance.

First, do not rush and don't be in a hurry to take up dance position. Smile, relax, give it some time and ease into it comfortably with your partner. Have some style, instead of just grabbing her.

It is always good to first do a couple of pulsing weight changes in place, left and right, to get into sync with the music and with your partner. You can also pulse and do some Charleston swivels in place to get into sync.

After this, you could for example do a couple of even walking steps or a couple of Pivot Turns before launching into the Balboa Basic or your first figure.

Another good start is to do a couple of Lollies simply from standing position, turning it into a Come-Around and there you are, right in the middle of dancing.

Always do simple moves initially, especially when dancing with a new partner. Increase the complexity gradually but not continuously. Return to simple moves once in a while.

Ending a dance when the music stops is easy enough as you can simply "stop dancing", i.e. finish the figure you are doing, slow down and let the dance fade out. This is perfectly fine, however, there are ways to make that ending feel more fun and look better.

For example, find figures that lend themselves to slowing down. Circular moves are better than linear ones. For example, it is easy to slow down Pivot Turns and come to a full stop in closed position. Or you can open up the follower into a side-by-side position, as if preparing for a pop Turn, and slow down and finish in that position.

The Slide is also a natural choice to mark the end of a song. It breaks the momentum of the dance and slows it down for the ending.

Correctly matching the ending move of the dance to the end of the song is important as it can look silly to make an ending move too early or too late.

Also, do not just leave your partner standing there and rush off to grab someone else when a dance is over. Thank her for the dance and escort her to her seat, unless she has other plans.

Dance floor conditions

How crowded the dance floor is will affect your dancing to some degree, although Balboa is designed specifically for crowded conditions.

It is primarily the leader's job to keep an eye on the surroundings. As you dance, guide your partner into the available space on the floor. Watch out for other dancers and keep away from those who dance recklessly or use large body movements. Your partner may sometimes look out for you and warn you of any danger behind you by pressing your hand or pulling you a little, but you cannot rely on her doing that.

The more crowded the floor the smaller you need to keep your dancing "footprint". In this case you may want to dance in close embrace only and limit your dancing to Pure Bal figures. Especially avoid backward movements as you cannot see who is behind you.

Although Balboa is not a progressive dance and you do not need to move around the dance floor, small collisions or bumps with other couples can happen. If they do, never make an issue of it and don't stop dancing. Apologize even if it was not your fault and move on smoothly.

Leaders and followers

Social dancing opens up never ending opportunities to meet, and dance with, a variety of new people. This comes with a few important consideration that are good to keep in mind.

First, since Balboa is a body-to-body dance, you will need to be somewhat mutually comfortable with a new dance partner. This is usually not an issue at a Balboa dance event because everyone will be aware of this. But when you try to dance Balboa at a Lindy Hop party, it is not always obvious whether your new dance partner is comfortable with this intimate dance position.

Further, when two strangers dance together for the first time, they both have some unspoken expectations relative to leading and following. What your new follower's particular expectations actually are you may never know, but generally speaking, what leaders want from followers and what followers want from leaders is not very complicated: Leaders want followers who know how to follow, and followers want leads who know how to lead.

Even more importantly, both leaders and followers hope to have a good time. At the end of the day, dancing is just a tool to have fun, and the goal should be to ensure that everyone is having fun, including you and your follower.

One of the best things one can do to maintain cordial relations is to refrain from teaching on the dance floor.

Teaching on the dance floor

Unsolicited teaching on the dance floor comes in two varieties and none of them is very productive. Version #1 is when you try to teach someone, and version #2 is when your dance partner is trying to teach you.

Often it is tempting to give advice to your dance partner for whatever reason (usually because you feel that she is not dancing very well). It is strongly recommended that you resist this temptation, even if you feel that you have the best of intentions.

Teaching someone means correcting her, and therefore it is a form of criticism. You may feel that you are doing a favour by sharing your wealth of knowledge, but she will simply feel that you are criticizing her. Guaranteed. Few people like to be criticised and they will feel irritated and confused even if they don't show it. After all, they came here to have fun, not to be put down.

Besides, it is also a very real possibility that when something is not working it is entirely your fault, not the follower's. If it is your fault, then you are really making a fool of yourself by trying to correct her. So the best approach is to dance your best, cover for her mistakes, and generally make the most of the experience.

Sometimes a follower will ask you to teach her. Again, it is recommended that you politely decline. Just say that you don't know her steps or that you are still learning this yourself. Teaching is a difficult art under the best of circumstances, but on the dance floor it is a messy, ineffective and hopeless business with the loud music blasting and all the people dancing around you. Anyone wanting to learn to dance is free to take some group lessons.

Receiving unsolicited advice from others, or asking others for advice, are similarly ineffective. However, you can still learn a lot by observing others dancing, taking notes of what you like, trying to break it down and practicing it on your own. It is also a good idea to ask people where they learned certain things, and then follow up on that trail.

The good follower

Followers come at all levels of experience. Sometimes a follower's level of experience will be obvious, but often you will not be able to judge it until you start dancing with her. For this reason, it is better to start every dance easy and to gradually increase the complexity of the steps you lead.

If it turns out that she is a beginner, it is best to dance at her level, to lead simple steps, let her practice what she already knows, and to focus on the social aspect of dancing with a new person.

Dancing with someone at your level (for example a current or former classmate) is generally ideal. It is great for practicing and gives a feeling of success to both parties.

If your partner is the better dancer, then use this as a learning opportunity, try some new steps and see how she reacts.

When dancing with someone, your own dancing will be affected by the weight, strength, timing and momentum of another body. This will be different with every follower, and with practice you need to develop a feel for how to adjust, adapt and compensate for this.

There are a few basic things a lead will generally hope for when dancing with a stranger.

The movement of the follower (just like yours) should be smooth and flexible, not rigid or jerky.

Even though the Balboa dance position requires a slight chest-to-chest pressure, the follower should generally keep her own balance, including during turns and spins, and not lean on the leader.

The follower should not grip your hand, as this prevents smooth adjustment of hand positions during turns or separations.

Assuming your lead is clear, a good follower will wait for and concentrate on the lead and not guess what figure is coming next. If she does guess, then she will often be wrong and dance something you are not leading at all.

Again assuming a clear lead, an experienced follower will quickly adjust to any unexpected moves you lead. She will react curiously and find an appropriate movement of her own, even if she never danced that step.

The partners will often leverage on each other through stretch and compression. The good follower is always ready to give you a solid but flexible frame. It is very difficult to lead a follower with "spaghetti arms".

During a free turn, the follower should keep her hand at approximately the same position where you released it, so that you can easily catch it again at the end of the turn. In most cases this will be at around waist level.

The good leader

Generally you cannot do much about how good a dancer your follower is, but you can do a lot about being a good leader yourself by practicing diligently and following a couple of rules of thumb.

Rule No. 1 for the leaders is: care about your follower and don't just dance for yourself.

You should also initiate every lead clearly and on time, without ambiguity or hesitation. The lead should be fluid and continuous, and the follower should never feel that the movement stops (unless the stop is deliberate).

"Calibrate" with your dance partner early on, assess her experience level and observe how she responds to certain moves.

If the follower does something else than what you expected her to do or tried to lead, never try to correct her. Go along, follow her, go with the flow and regain control.

Being a show-off generally does not contribute to being a good leader. On the other hand, if your objective is to make your partner look good and feel good, it is virtually guaranteed that you will be a sought-after dancer. The rule of thumb is: if the follower is smiling, you are doing fine.

But even if you do everything well, you will never be a perfect lead for everyone because each follower has different expectations, likes and dislikes.